Li[illegible] to

•••••••••

Three studies of health and well-being among older people in East London and Essex

Ann Bowling, Emily Grundy
and Morag Farquhar

AGE Concern

BOOKS

Age Concern England is pleased to offer customised editions of all its titles to UK companies, institutions or other organisations wishing to make a bulk purchase. For further information please contact the Publishing Department at the address on this page.
Tel: 0181-679 8000. Fax: 0181-679 6069. Email: addisom@ace.org.uk

Published by Age Concern England
1268 London Road
London SW16 4ER

First published 1997

Designed and typeset by GreenGate Publishing Services, Tonbridge, Kent
Printed in Great Britain by Bell & Bain Ltd., Glasgow

A catalogue record for this book is available from the British Library
ISBN 0-86242-243-4

Contents

About the authors

Ann Bowling, a sociologist, is currently Professor of Health Services Research at University College London Medical School. Her research on ageing includes evaluation of developments in care interfaces and work on measuring the quality of life.

Emily Grundy, a demographer, is a Reader in Social Gerontology at King's College London. Apart from her research, which focuses on intergenerational relationships, household, and health in older age groups, her work includes teaching on the Institute's MSc in Gerontology programme.

Morag Farquhar, who did much of the interviewing on which this book is based, has recently had a second baby and is currently having a career break. She lives in Essex.

Acknowledgements

We are grateful to the many interviewers, coding, administrative and research staff who have contributed to this project, in particular Lesley Marriott, Juliet Formby and Ganka Mueller, and to the respondents who made the study possible. We are also grateful to staff at the Office for National Statistics (formerly the Office of Population Censuses and Surveys) for flagging the death entries, to Dr Jane Leaver for her on-going enthusiasm and support, and to other members of the advisory group for their advice.

The baseline studies were funded by City and Hackney Health Authority and Mid-Essex Health Authority. The Joseph Rowntree Foundation funded the longitudinal follow-up study reported on here.

Our thanks also go to Jane Brotchie, Words in Action, Brighton for her invaluable editorial help.

The Joseph Rowntree Foundation has supported this project as part of its programme of research and innovative development projects, which it hopes will be of value to policy makers and practitioners. The facts presented and views expressed in this report, however, are those of the authors and not necessarily those of the Foundation.

Introduction

In 1949, a report from the Royal Commission on Population suggested that a society with a falling proportion of young people might become 'dangerously unprogressive, falling behind other communities not only in technical efficiency and economic welfare but in artistic and intellectual achievement as well'. Few contemporary commentators would so readily dismiss the contribution of older people to the well-being of society. But the increasingly old population is still perceived as a major challenge. Will longer life and increasing numbers of older people be a burden or a boon?

This book explores the concept of 'successful' survival in old age and presents the results of research conducted over three years with older people in Hackney in Inner London and Braintree in Essex. Over 1,000 people were interviewed and the views of older people themselves have informed the design and recommendations that emerge from this study.

The aim of the research was initially to gather information on the health, well-being and social support of older populations in Hackney and Essex. Follow-up interviews, funded by the Rowntree Foundation, enabled the research to expand its aims to document and analyse changes in the ability to manage tasks of daily living, physical health, mental health, service use and social circumstances. The data offers new evidence, not only about the difficulties of old age, but also about the factors that contribute to well-being and to experiencing a 'good old age'.

The structure of the book

Chapter 1 *What is 'successful' ageing?* This chapter discusses the ambivalent attitudes we currently hold towards ageing in our society. It explores some of the conceptual difficulties of 'successful' ageing and suggests that neutral terms such as 'well-being' and 'quality of life' might be more appropriate.

Chapter 2 *The research study* This chapter explains the background to the research and how the study was designed to yield information about well-being and quality of life for older people.

Chapter 3 *Well-being in old age in Hackney and Braintree* Here, we present the main results from the study concerning the physical and mental well-being of older people and the changes that occurred over the two to three year interval between interviews.

Chapter 4 *What sustains well-being and quality of life in the oldest old?* This chapter explores what sets apart those who are experiencing a 'good old age' from those with multiple problems and looks at changes in the situation of very old people on a range of dimensions.

Chapter 5 *Implications for policy development and service delivery* We suggest some ways in which services could be developed to enable more older people to enjoy a happy and active old age.

1 *What is successful ageing?*

• Longer life: gift or burden?

It is no longer news to say we live in an ageing population. People are living longer and the proportion of people over 85 is increasing. The long-term decline in birth rates mean that those in older age categories comprise a larger share of the total population than in the past. The essential question is whether we regard this development as a threat to our collective welfare or as an opportunity for greater life fulfilment. Are the 'extra years', which more of us can now look forward to, going to be really enjoyable – or will they be marred by poor health and social isolation?

Living longer means more people can look forward to a life beyond work and child rearing. Yet ambivalence about our older and still ageing, population remains. This ambivalence reflects a number of negative assumptions and fears.

A time of decline and dependency?

Ageist stereotypes of older people persist; many regard ageing as a negative experience – a time of decline, illness and disability. Older people continue to be described as a burden on society. Changes in patterns of family organisation, such as the rise of divorce and the number of single parents, have further fuelled fears that younger generations may not be able to meet the needs of the old, although evidence of this is far from clear cut. Family support is sometimes thought to be dwindling in comparison with a largely mythical 'lost world' where all old people supposedly lived in the bosom of their families, revered by all until they did the decent thing and died at three score years and ten.

How will we meet the costs?

There are, of course, valid reasons for concern. Policy makers are alarmed by the prospect of the rising costs of health care and pensions needed to support more older people over a longer period of time. Government estimates of per capita public health and personal social service expenditure in 1989–90 show the figures for those over 85 years to be 15 times as great as expenditure on those aged 15–64 and four and a half times as great as expenditure on 65–74-year-olds.

The Gerontological Society of America in the first issue of the *Journal of Gerontology*, published 50 years ago, adopted the slogan 'adding life to years' rather than years to life. How to do this is the question that continues to interest both researchers and practitioners. The challenge is to identify the risks of old age and to find ways of reducing them, so that more people can experience 'a good old age'. Concepts such as 'successful' or 'positive' ageing are increasingly used, but these rather loose terms have a range of meanings, partly depending on a person's background. For example, those involved in public health stress the importance of staying physically and mentally fit, psychologists see 'successful' ageing as the ability to adapt to changing circumstances, and sociologists equate 'success' with strong feelings of satisfaction with life.

Responses from men and women aged 75 to 95 from Hackney and Essex

'Health and decent homes come first.'

'We need companionship, company is the most important thing I think … somebody to talk to … to tell jokes … '

'Services are very important for people who can't get out. We are the lucky ones that can get out.'

'We've all been robbed and mugged … that's not making us happy is it?'

'Somebody to call on if you are taken bad or fall down – someone you can rely on.'

'Knowing someone is there to help … because then you can help yourself. You have to be able to adapt.'

'Having nothing wrong with you … being able to do things, but with arthritis everything gets worse … '

'Being able to keep your end up … not giving in, waiting for *the* telegram.'

Previously published in *MRC News*, 1994

A happy old age

What does a 'good old age' mean? Older people who participated in discussion groups during the research gave their views.

As the comments in the box suggest, there are several factors that are commonly associated with a good old age. Among them are: staying fit, maintaining social contact, and having some choice in where to live and who you live with. Below, we briefly review what current research tells us about each of these topics.

• Staying fit in later life

From a medical point of view, 'successful' ageing is achieving a long life expectancy, while at the same time delaying the onset of infirmity, so that illness is compressed into a shorter period. Biological limitations cannot be ignored but quality of life in old age can be improved by the flexible and positive adaptation of the individual and by early intervention or prevention strategies to slow down a decline in functional ability.

Most people aged 65 and over are able to perform all tasks of daily living unaided, albeit sometimes with a degree of difficulty. However, the prevalence of long-standing illness is high in older age groups. The *OPCS Disability Survey* (Martin *et al.*, 1988) in the UK reported that the prevalence of severe disability was 133 per 1,000 for people aged 80 years and over, compared with 16 per 1,000 for people in their sixties and three per 1,000 for adults aged under 50. Women have a longer life expectancy than men, but they are likely to spend a longer time disabled.

The common problems

The *OPCS Disability Survey* emphasised the high prevalence in old age of disabilities affecting hearing, sight and mobility. The most common causes of long-standing illness among people aged 75 and over, as reported in the General Household Survey in Britain, are arthritis and rheumatism, other bone and joint problems, cataracts, hypertension, heart attack and other heart problems.

Improving well-being, reducing infirmity

Chronic illnesses do not necessarily result in disability. Some have argued that dependency is exacerbated by the organisation and expectations of society. Osteoarthritis, for example, may be a disabling condition, but much can be done to organise the home to make life easier and to keep the sufferer mobile. In some cases, the condition can be largely remedied through prosthetic intervention. Ease of access to transport in the immediate environment also affects a person's ability to get about.

Individual ability to adapt

Psycho-social, as well as physical factors, influence the outcomes of impairment. Thus, how a person feels about their illness or impairment and how ready they are to adapt to change can also be important.

The single most common psychiatric diagnosis among community samples of older people is depression. Risk factors for depression include poor health, bereavement, lack of companionship, economic deprivation and, to a lesser extent, age. Women are also more likely than men to be depressed.

Life satisfaction

Under the broader umbrella of psycho-social adjustment, the achievement of high life satisfaction has been identified, along with physical health status, as an essential dimension of 'successful' ageing.

Studies in the USA and across Europe have shown that the most consistent and strongest associations with life satisfaction are how individuals rate their own state of health (perceived health status), their ability to carry out tasks of daily life (functional ability) and level of income.

• Maintaining social contact

In the 1960s the 'disengagement' model of ageing was popular. Social scientists suggested that older people gradually relinquished social roles in preparation for death and that this process benefited both the older person and society as a whole. This model has now been largely superseded by 'activity' theories which stress the importance of maintaining social interaction and substituting new roles or relationships for those lost.

Many studies have shown that the more social ties a person carries into middle or old age, the healthier they are likely to stay. Research in the United States suggests that social contact stimulates the body's immune responses which keep us healthy. Those who have a network of family or friends are more likely to have help with daily activities when needed, which is likely to lead to better nutrition and hygiene. Such social support is thought to be particularly important as a buffer against stress, an important factor since later life involves potentially stressful changes such as bereavement and illnesses.

• Living alone and living with others in old age

In the developed world, recent decades have seen large increases in the proportion of older people living by themselves, half of all those over 75 now live alone. This is often viewed in a negative light, but all indications show that older people value their independence and, in the main, live alone because more are now able to do so. Results from the Eurobarometer Survey by the European Commission show that it is in Greece, where a large proportion of older people live with their younger relatives, that the reported prevalence of loneliness and poor life satisfaction is the highest. In the Nordic countries, where living alone is more common, reported loneliness is lower.

Choices and constraints

Higher incomes and a greater availability of suitable housing have enabled more older people to purchase the privacy they desire. 'Intimacy at a distance' appears to be the preferred option for older people and their families.

Of course, not all older people have benefited from increased *choice* in living arrangements. Constraints on both living arrangements and residential mobility may in some cases be a more important consideration. The most obvious example is the constraint of kin availability on household patterns – childless widows cannot choose to live with spouses and children.

Poor health may also reduce choices for those who develop substantial support needs and who lack sufficient assistance inside or outside the home. For some, options may be limited to moving in with a relative or entering an institution.

Other obvious constraints are income and availability of suitable housing. Nearly all the older people in Hackney included in this study had low incomes and only a small minority owned their own homes. Although many said they would like to move, clearly their ability to do so was limited.

Living arrangements often change with advancing age. While the vast majority of 'young' older people live alone or in nuclear families, among the older old, aged 85 and over, quite high proportions live either in institutions or with relatives.

Living alone – a health risk?

Most studies indicate that old people who live with relatives have poorer health than those living alone: this is largely because poor health is often a reason for moving to live with a relative or being joined by a relative. Living arrangements may also directly influence health. Although most studies suggest that those living alone are not an 'at risk' group and the literature overwhelmingly indicates that living alone and loneliness should not be confused, there are some indications that among men, if not women, living alone may be associated with poor psycho-social and general health. Apart from lack of emotional support within the household, an absence of practical support may have negative effects on the health of older men who live alone. US studies, for example, suggest that they have a poorer diet.

Confusion over the causal associations between health and household status is evident in policy. Despite repeated demands that services should be targetted on families caring for old people with high support needs, those living alone still receive far more assistance from formal health and welfare providers.

• Who defines 'success'?

While there may be some general consensus about the factors that contribute to 'successful' ageing, the concept is itself problematic. Many definitions of 'successful' ageing suffer from being tautological or involve reference to similarly vague or poorly defined concepts, including health. Definitions of 'success' also imply a norm or value system that may not be appropriate. Roos and Harevens (1991) for example, suggested that remaining outside an institution without continuing support services indicated 'successful' ageing. However, if people living in the community have unmet needs for assistance this might be regarded as failure. Partly for these reasons. we prefer to use neutral concepts, such as 'quality of life' or 'well-being', rather than terms such as 'successful' or 'positive' ageing.

2 *The research study*

This chapter gives some background to the study as a whole and explains how the research was designed and carried out.

• Strengths and limitations of the study

The strength of this study is the information it provides about *changing* circumstances. The research is based on a two- to three-year follow-up study of the health and well-being of three samples of older people: over 1,000 people in total. The large sample size is unusual – data on the 85+ age group is especially sparse in Britain. The *1985 General Household Survey* for example – which had a special section on older people – only included some 250 respondents aged 85 and over.

A limitation of the study is that it is, by definition, about those people living in the community (outside institutions), which, with the 85+ age group, inevitably means that the least healthy are excluded. Moreover, the study of course embraces only survivors who, in the case of those in the 85+ sample, comprise only a minority of their birth group.

• Cohort (generational) differences

This study concerns people born between the late 1880s and the early 1920s. As shown in Figures la and 1b the chances of survival to old age were substantially greater for those born later in this period. Those in

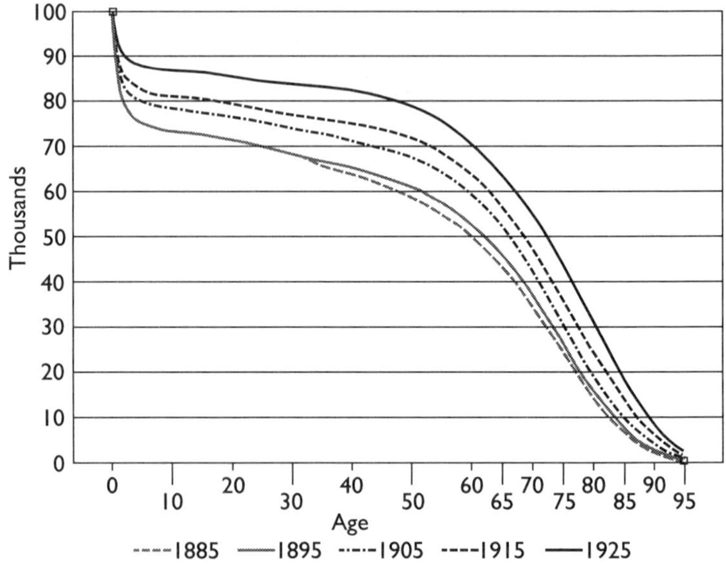

Figure 1a Male survivorship by year of birth: England and Wales
(Source: Government Actuary's Department)

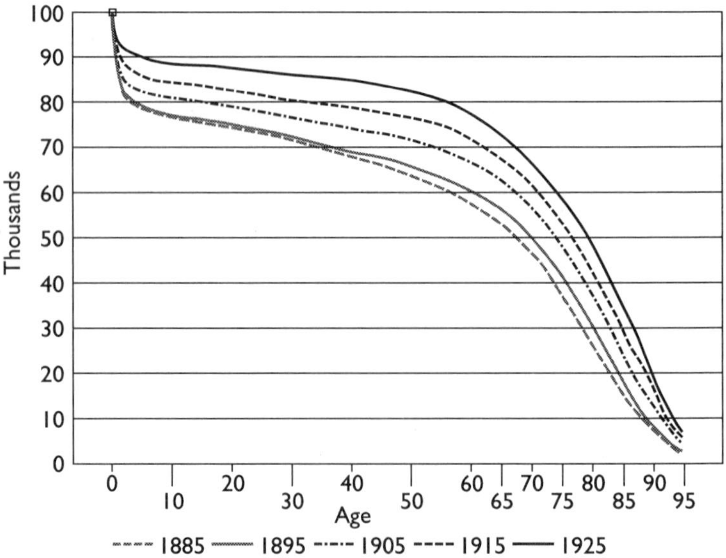

Figure 1b Female survivorship by year of birth: England and Wales

our oldest sample, who were aged 85 or over when first interviewed in 1987, represent only a small proportion of their birth cohort, many of whom failed to survive to adulthood, let alone advanced old age. This raises a number of questions about how far their characteristics reflect their special 'survivor' status and how far the characteristics of later generations, with better survival prospects, will differ.

Is a good old age predetermined in earlier life?

It is evident that people reach old age with certain aspects of their life already fixed. For example, the number of children they have had and, in nearly all cases, their formal education. These prior events, lifestyles and inheritances (all of which are both genetic and environmental) are known to be important influences on health in later life. Disentangling the effects of earlier life from current or recent influences is not possible from our research because it is confined to data collected from people who have already reached old age. But what the research *can* show, because of its longitudinal design, is the extent of change within old age.

• Who was included in the surveys?

The three surveys were:

- a survey of 630 people aged 85 or more who lived in Hackney
- two parallel studies of 'younger' old people – 65–84 year olds – in Hackney and Braintree.

The samples were drawn from contrasting areas: Hackney in Inner London and Braintree in Essex. Hackney is an inner-city area with more than its share of inner-city problems. It had high scores on indices of deprivation based on the 1981 and 1991 Censuses.

The mid-Essex area, centred on Braintree is, by contrast, a relatively prosperous semi-rural area. Of course, attributing the characteristics of areas to the people resident there represents an 'ecological fallacy': that is, not all people in poor and deprived areas are necessarily poor and deprived. It is particularly important to remember this when the population of older people is being considered, as most of them were born or settled in their current locality many decades ago.

The follow-up work, funded by the Rowntree Foundation, included re-interviews with surviving sample members some two to three years after the first survey, together with the tracing of deaths (via the National Health Services Central Register) and some follow up of service use. In summary, the data set consists of the following elements:

Table 1

Baseline surveys	Follow-up surveys	Other follow up
Hackney, 630* persons aged 85+ (1987) (Born 1886–1902)	Re-interviews with 263 survivors (1990: Jan–June)	Tracing of deaths, hospital admissions; entry long-term care
Hackney, 464 persons aged 65–84 (1989) (Born 1904–1924)	Re-interviews with 330 survivors (1991 Feb–July)	Tracing of deaths, hospital admissions entry long-term care
Mid-Essex, 276 persons aged 65–84 (1989) (Born 1904–1924)	Re-interviews with 195 survivors (1991: April–August)	Tracing of deaths, hospital admissions, entry long-term care; use of services

*10 of these were subsequently found not to have reached their 85th birthday at the baseline interview and have been excluded from some analyses.

Samples and response rates

The 85+ study in Hackney included the whole population in this age range living in the City and Hackney Health District area. The other two groups were representative random samples of people aged 65–85. Family Practitioner Committee (now Family Health Service Area) records were cross checked against the electoral register and other sources, and were used to identify the population to be sampled. The research design was approved by the relevant ethical committees and the aims of the research were explained to all participants.

The initial (baseline) survey of the 85+ sample in Hackney gave a 70 per cent response rate. with the follow-up survey having a 78 per cent response rate. The 65–85-year-old samples had response rates of 67 per cent in Hackney and 82 per cent in Braintree. The response rates for the follow-up surveys were 82 per cent in Hackney and 77 per cent in Braintree.

Characteristics of sample members

Table 2 shows the age and sex distribution of the three samples at first interview. The Braintree sample was younger than the equivalent Hackney sample; this largely reflects the different age composition of the population of older people in these areas. However, the under-representation of men in the Braintree sample cannot be attributed to this. Investigation showed that men in Braintree were just as likely as women to agree to take part in the study, so this anomaly seems to be due to 'sampling error': that is, it is a reflection of the fact that we interviewed a sample rather than the whole population. In comparison with the equivalent Hackney group, more of those in Braintree were married and far fewer were single (never married); this partly reflects the different age structure of the two groups.

Table 2 Distribution of the baseline samples by age and sex (%)

Age group	Braintree 65–84			Hackney 65–84			Hackney 85+		
	Men	Women	Total	Men	Women	Total	Men	Women	Total
65–74	63	60	61	54	40	46	–	–	
75–84	37	40	39	46	60	54	–	–	
85–89	–	–	–	–	–	–	79	73	74
90+	–	–	–	–	–	–	21	27	26
Total %	100	100	100	100	100	100	100	100	100
N	87	183	270	186	268	454	136	484	620
% Female			68			59			78

Table 3 shows the housing and household characteristics of the baseline samples. Most of the older people interviewed in Hackney lived in flats and some two thirds were council tenants. Only just over ten per

Table 3 Household and housing characteristics of samples at baseline (%)

	Braintree 65–84	Hackney 65–84	Hackney 85+
Housing tenure			
Local authority tenant	41	69	63
Private tenant	7	11	12
Owner-occupier	48	11	12
Other	4	9	12
Housing type			
Flat	16	82	82
House/bungalow	83	15	15
Other	1	3	3
Household size			
1	36	55	61
2	54	34	29
3+	10	11	10

cent owned their houses, and an equivalent proportion lived in accommodation rented from private landlords. In Braintree, by contrast, nearly half the sample were owner-occupiers and most lived in houses or bungalows. The proportion living alone was also much lower in Braintree than in Hackney: a difference largely due to the higher proportion who were married. As Figure 2 shows, the proportion of single (never-married) people was much lower in Braintree than in Hackney, as was the proportion widowed. Most of the 85+ group were widowed at the time of the baseline survey and by the time of the follow-up survey the proportion widowed had increased further; the same was true of the younger samples.

The difference in the age structure of the 65–84-year-old Hackney and Braintree samples may influence other results, such as differences in marital or health status. Similarly, many of the characteristics we were interested in, such as life satisfaction, physical and mental health, are interrelated. In order to disentangle these qualities, we undertook a range of multivariate statistical analyses. These analyses are not presented in this book, but the results we report here are based on this more complex statistical analysis. A list of the published papers arising

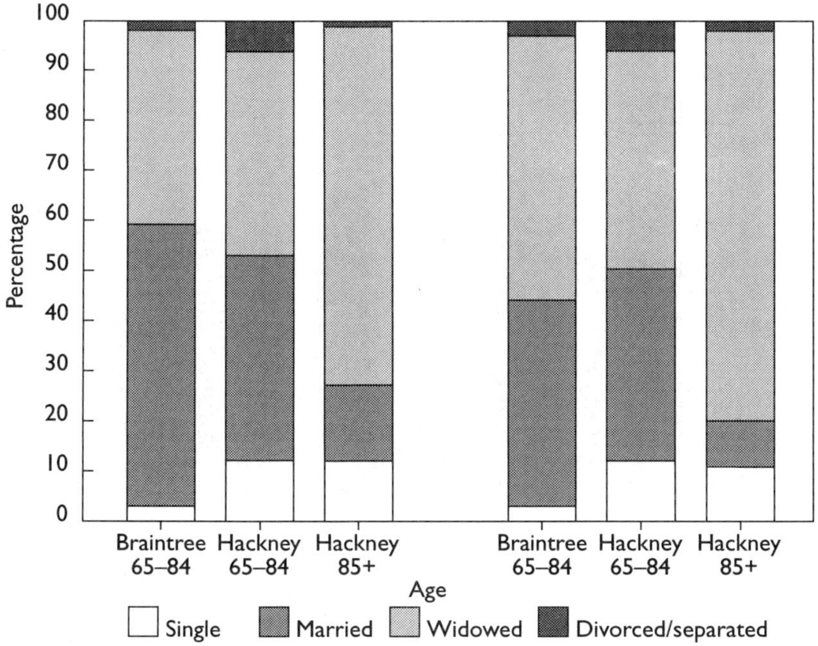

Figure 2 Distribution at baseline and follow-up stage of males and females in Essex and Hackney by marital status

from the study, in which more details of the work done may be found, is given in Appendix 2.

The results of this research relate to local samples; in Figures 3a and 3b we have compared some of our results with the national sample included in the *1985 General Household Survey*. Our oldest old Hackney sample was very similar to the national one with regard to the prevalence of mobility and self-care limitations, the proportion of people living alone, the proportion of females and the proportion unmarried. However, a much higher proportion of the older population in Hackney were local authority tenants. While this is partly a reflection of post-war reconstruction and slum-clearance programmes in this area, it is also an indication of the lower socio-economic status of the sample compared with the population as a whole.

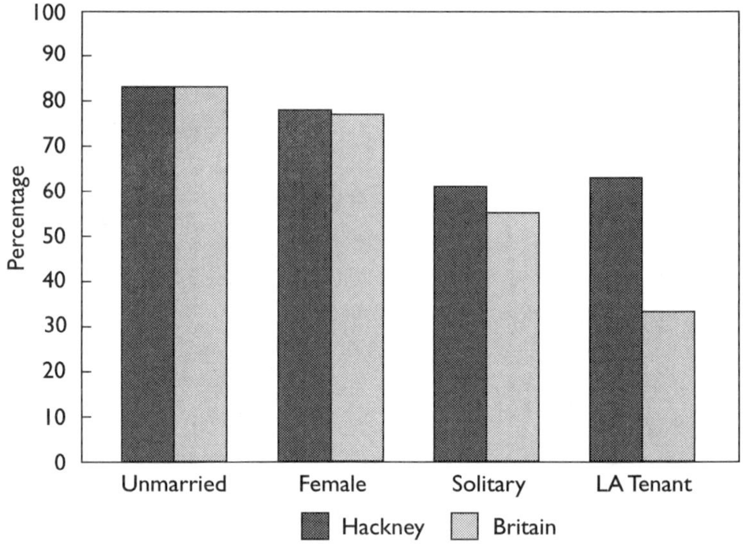

Figure 3a Comparison of Hackney 85+ sample with national sample; socio-demographic characteristics

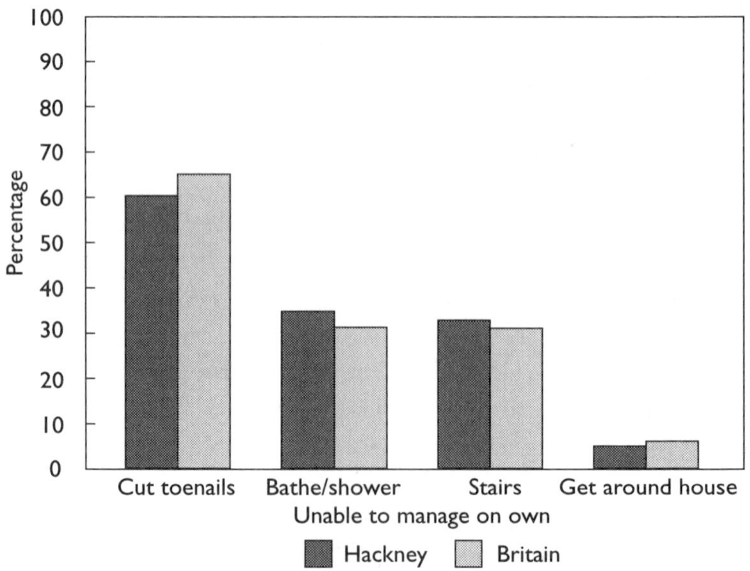

Figure 3b Comparison of Hackney sample with national sample; mobility and self-care

• Measuring well-being and quality of life

As discussed in Chapter 1, the concept of 'successful' ageing is problematic, which makes translating it into a measurable quality a difficult task. Baltes and Baltes (1990) identified a number of indicators which feature strongly in the literature of 'successful' ageing. These were: length of life, biological health, mental health, cognitive efficacy, social competence and personal control over circumstances and life satisfaction. They suggested that the key was 'selective optimisation with compensation' – in other words, the ability to make the most of personal strengths and develop strategies to cope with weaknesses.

Although the literature on 'successful' or 'positive' ageing has principally been written by contributors from the behavioural and social sciences, many of the key indicators identified – such as the ability to undertake activities of daily living, physical health and mental health – have long formed the kernel of multi-dimensional assessments of the health and well-being of older people.

The studies in Hackney and Essex featured here, were based on a concept of health that is broader than one focused on disease, or the absence of disease. We gathered information on social, psychological and environmental circumstances as well as looking at, for example, changes in the physical functioning of study members. By following up individuals after two or three years, we were able to document and analyse changes in:

- ability to undertake activities of daily living
- physical health
- anxiety and depression
- service use
- social circumstances.

As well as looking at changes in these domains and seeing how they were associated with other factors, we also wanted to look at well-being over a range of indicators to build a multidimensional picture of 'quality of life'. How many old people had multiple problems and difficulties and how many had none or few? To do this we looked at how many 'good' or 'poor' scores respondents had in the various important domains of life.

Scales measuring psychiatric morbidity (the incidence of depression and anxiety), life satisfaction, degree of difficulty with activities of daily living, social support, and other main variables (health symptoms, service use, etc) were selected after a careful review of the relevant literature. (These scales are described in more detail in Appendix 1.)

After focused group discussions with older people about factors they felt were important for a happy old age, and a further review of relevant literature, we identified variables that together would provide an indication of quality of life. This process led us to select variables for analysis which represent three domains of life: perceived well-being (life satisfaction), health and activity, and environment.

We wished to consider in more detail those at the 'top' and 'bottom' end of the continuum with a view to identifying factors that may predispose people towards the enjoyment of a 'good old age', or its inverse.

Having selected our variables, the next step was to investigate the pattern of their interdependence and to develop a composite measure of well-being. This enabled us to identify the proportion of men and women with 'good' and 'poor' scores and to look at changes in the distribution of the sample according to the responses to these items.

THREE AREAS CHOSEN TO INDICATE QUALITY OF LIFE AND WELL-BEING

The following variables were chosen to analyse the results of the data.

Perceived well-being

- Life satisfaction score
- Perceived control and autonomy

Health and Activity

- Score on a measure of ability to undertake activities of daily living
- Health problems from a checklist of ten common complaints
- Anxiety and depression as measured on the General Health Questionnaire
- A 'usual activities' question on time spent 'doing nothing, just sitting'

Environment

- Whether the respondent had fears about opening the door, intruders or going out
- Whether the respondent liked the area he or she lived in
- Whether the respondent's home was warm enough (this was only used in the 85+ study).

The importance of environment

While indicators of health and life satisfaction are very much the staple fare of studies of old people, environmental factors are less routinely considered. We would suggest that they are an important component of overall 'quality of life', not only directly but also as an indicator of socio-economic status.

Fears for personal safety were a dominant theme in the group discussions and were felt to be a major constraint on activities, so a question about these fears was also included. Respondents were also asked whether or not they liked the area in which they lived.

3 *Well-being in old age in Hackney and Braintree*

This chapter presents the key research findings. They are listed under the following headings: mental well-being, physical well-being, the social ties and use of services, differences in survival and quality of life. The chapter concludes with a discussion about some of the characteristics that appear to be associated with successful survival in the community.

• Mental well-being

The surveys measured two aspects of mental well-being:

- anxiety and depression (measured by the General Health Questionnaire (GHQ)
- life satisfaction.

Anxiety and depression

In our study, one of the most striking findings was the importance of physical health for mental health. Anxiety and depression were consistently associated with poor health and persistently poor, or deteriorating, levels of functional ability. Conversely, improvements in health and functioning were associated with improvements in mental health.

Anxiety and depression were more common in the oldest group (see Table 4) and more common among women than men. Deterioration in mental health (anxiety and depression) was also greatest amongst the 85+ sample, with about a quarter of people aged 85 and over suffering symptoms. By follow-up time, almost one-fifth of this older sample with no previous symptoms had developed symptoms of anxiety and depression, and almost as many remained anxious and depressed over both interviewing periods. These changes are shown in Figure 4.

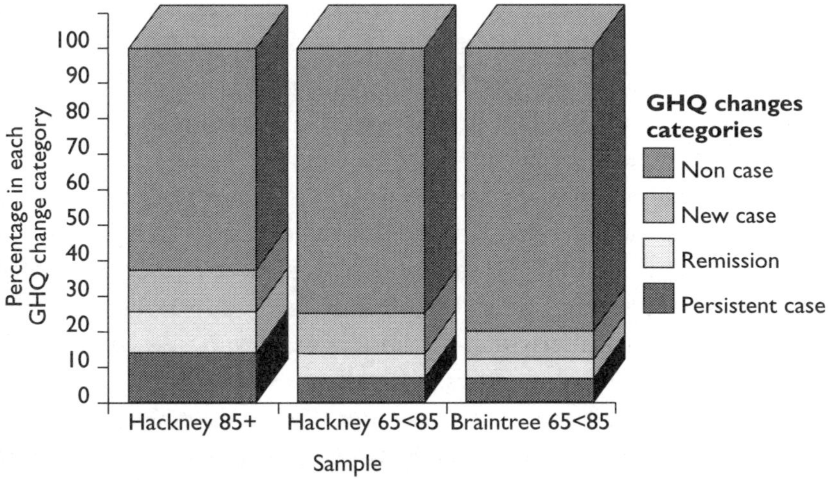

Figure 4 Changes in GHQ score between baseline and follow-up stage

Medical intervention appeared to be low, given the high rate of reported symptoms suggesting clinical depression. Very few older people who were depressed were receiving any form of antidepressant medication. (Interviewers inspected and noted details of all medication taken by respondents; this information was coded by a pharmacist using the British National Formulary classification.) The proportion of older people who reported physical symptoms and sleeplessness to their GP was high, but there was more reluctance to consult the GP for mental confusion and other psychosomatic symptoms, such as loss of appetite and forgetfulness.

Analyses described more fully elsewhere (see Appendix 2) showed that other factors associated with anxiety and depression included lower numbers of relatives in the social network, lower level of daily contact with relatives, friends or neighbours and greater feelings of loneliness.

Life satisfaction

A further measure of mental health, life satisfaction, was also examined at the initial interview and at the follow-up. Life satisfaction means an assessment of an individual's life, or a comparison, reflecting some perceived discrepancy between one's aspirations and achievement. Instruments assessing life satisfaction are increasing in popularity among researchers, partly in order to shift the focus from negative aspects of health to the more positive aspects. (For further information on the life satisfaction scales used in this research refer to Appendix 1.)

Poor and worsening life satisfaction was most clearly associated with some worsening ability to perform everyday tasks and with health status, particularly among those aged 85 and over. Between 27 and 32 per cent of the members of the three samples had poor overall life satisfaction at the first interview. These proportions hardly changed over time, although, as shown in Figure 5, some individuals improved or deteriorated.

Although social networks were not the strongest predicting factor in life satisfaction scores, there were notable differences in the social networks of those who reported a change in life satisfaction. Those who were 85 and over with poor life satisfaction at both initial and follow-up interview, were most likely to have the fewest relatives, friends and confidants. The density of networks was also important; density refers to the degree to which network members are in touch with each other. Those with poor life satisfaction tended to have the smallest network density at the initial interview and at follow-up. Losses in the number of friends was associated with worsening life satisfaction among the 85+ group.

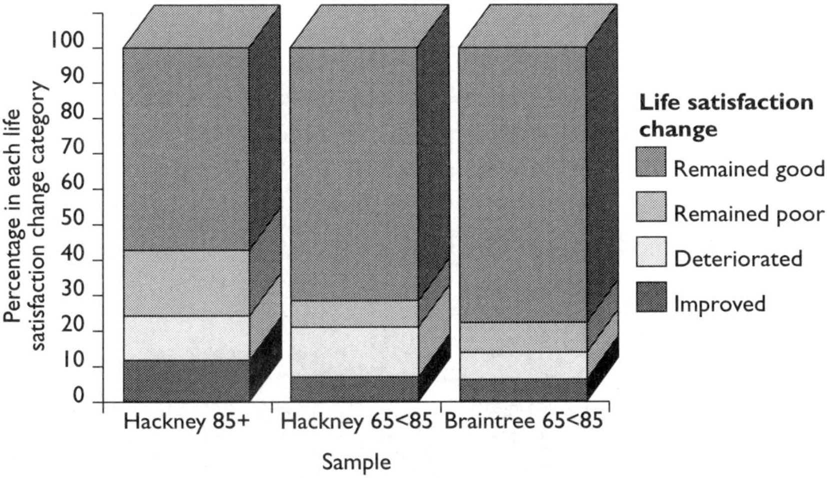

Figure 5 Changes in life satisfaction score in all three samples between baseline and follow up

Physical well-being

Physical health problems

Other studies, such as the *OPCS Disability Surveys*, have shown that problems with feet are, not surprisingly, a major cause of mobility difficulties among older people. We also found that problems with feet were most consistently associated with a decline in overall ability to cope with everyday living. Those who showed an improvement over time in their general level of functioning were less likely to have problems with their feet.

Other difficulties that were often reported were problems with nerves, bronchitis, sleeplessness, appetite loss, headache, chest pain and giddiness and – particularly with the 85+ sample – aches and pains in muscles and joints. Among the 85+ group, there were also problems with poor eyesight, even when wearing glasses, and with poor hearing, even when wearing a hearing aid. The high prevalence of musculoskeletal, eyesight and hearing problems found among this group of very old people is consistent with results from other surveys.

Changes in ability to perform activities of daily living

As would be expected, more of the oldest group had high functional disability scores at baseline (see Table 4 – p 35) and deterioration was also associated with increasing age. For example, while one-fifth of the 85+ sample deteriorated, just 12 per cent and eight per cent respectively of the younger 65–85 Hackney and Braintree samples deteriorated. Figure 6 illustrates these changes for the three samples.

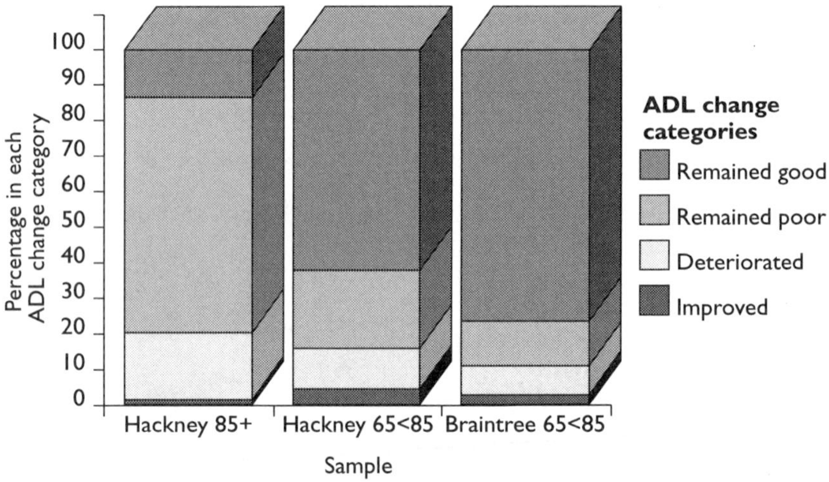

Figure 6 Changes in ADL score between baseline and follow up in all three samples between baseline and follow up

As reported previously, the single physical health symptom which was consistently associated with chronic difficulties in daily living was trouble with feet. High scores indicating anxiety and depression were also consistently associated with chronic difficulties and with deterioration over time.

Women were more likely to report such difficulties than men, although this was partly due to the older age composition of the female group. There were also some differences according to where respondents lived. For example, the Hackney sample had a poorer ability to perform everyday tasks than the equivalent Braintree sample.

In the 85+ group, ability to perform tasks of daily living was associated with changes in living arrangements. Nearly one-third of women living alone at the first interview who had severe problems with several aspects of daily living were in institutions by the time of the follow-up interview.

Difficulties getting out

If older people are to live independently in the community they need to be able to get out of doors. Few respondents aged 65–84 reported that they were housebound, but the proportion increased to 45 per cent among respondents aged 85 or over at initial interview. One half of those people aged 85 or over with no difficulties getting out of doors at initial interview had deteriorated by the time of their follow-up interview.

Coping with daily living

Tasks which respondents particularly noted as having some degree of difficulty involved were: using public transport, cutting toenails, climbing stairs/steps, laundry, getting about outdoors, getting in and out of the bath and filling in forms/writing.

The activities which the largest proportions of respondents reported experiencing severe difficulty with, or could not do at all were: odd jobs around the home (including changing light bulbs and fuses, gardening and window cleaning), using public transport, shopping, handling money/their pension, and cutting toenails.

Those who had severe difficulties with going out, or who could not go out at all, had poorer mental health and life satisfaction and reported experiencing more problems and pain with activities of daily living than other groups.

Among the 85+ group, the most consistent associations between inability to get around outside and with health problems were with eyesight (even when wearing glasses) and with aches, pain and/or stiffness in muscles and joints.

Not surprisingly, there were significant associations between ability to get around out of doors and involvement in social activities. While most respondents in the older age group said that they regularly or occasionally watched television and listened to the radio, and between two-thirds and three-quarters said that they read books, magazines or newspapers, far fewer engaged in more active pursuits. Many activities depend on the ability to go outside the home. Those who could not go out alone were reliant on another person's help to take them out, and those who could not get out, even with help, were totally excluded from these activities. One example is shopping or 'window shopping', which was an activity a number of those who were housebound said they missed.

Ability to get outside also has an effect on a person's relationships with others, because inability to get out easily means that it is impossible to visit relatives, neighbours and friends. Older people confined to the house become more reliant on having visitors.

Table 4 Percentage of respondents with health limitations at baseline

	Braintree		Hackney		
	65–74	**75–84**	**65–74**	**75–84**	**85+**
Reported 5+ health problems	16	17	27	37	45
GHQ score 6+	11	18	10	21	26
Poor functional ability (score 71+)	3	11	7	14	41
Cannot get out of doors or has severe difficulty getting out of doors	5	17	9	21	51

• Social ties and use of services

Contrary to popular images of very old people as lonely or isolated, most respondents were found to be well supported by their families and friends. Very few older respondents lacked any emotional and social ties. Loss of relatives, friends and confidants was greatest, as would be expected, in the 85+ sample. Most people had at least one person in their social networks, although 14 per cent of very old people in the Hackney sample had no one in their networks by the time of the follow-up interview. At the time of both interviews, relatives provided a great deal of help with most activities of daily living in all three samples; friends provided little help. Professionals helped with odd jobs, personal care tasks, such as cutting toenails. Table 5 (p 38) shows what proportions of the Hackney 85+ survivors needed help with particular tasks at the time of the follow-up interview and who provided that help. At this stage, most of these very old people needed help with shopping, housework and laundry. A lower proportion reported needing help with cooking, but this probably partly reflects the fact that most of them received meals on wheels. Professionals helped with housework more often than relatives, and, as noted above, also predominated among those helping with cutting toenails, but help with shopping and laundry was as likely to be provided by a relative as a professional. Help with filling in forms and odd jobs was usually provided by relatives.

Carers of very old people may suffer increased strain over time because the size of a person's network is characterised by a decreasing number of relatives as the person grows older, so care falls on a smaller number of people. This study showed that while network size declined, and one-third of the 85+ group reported having fewer relatives in their networks, there was little change in the proportion who could name a main helper. This finding give further weight to the demands for more help and support for family carers.

These results are based on the samples chosen for this study which, by definition, included only those old people who were living in the community. An earlier survey of older people (65 and over) on waiting lists for institutional care in the City and Hackney showed that 23 per cent had no regular contact with relatives, friends or neighbours (Bowling 1989). This would seem to support previous work suggesting that supportive networks enable very old people to remain living in the community.

Use of other services such as district nursing and home help services, was clearly associated with frailty – in other words, those who were most frail were in receipt of most services. However, the services that were being used tended to be 'maintenance' rather than preventive. Use of formal services was heavier in the inner city, older people living in Hackney used more services than those in Braintree. Few respondents in any groups used carer relief services or preventive and rehabilitation services such as occupational therapy or physiotherapy.

At both the initial and follow-up interviews about four-fifths of the sample members reported having been to see their general practitioners in the last 12 months. Those with poorer levels of functioning were less likely to have been in contact with opticians and dentists.

Unmet need

Few of the Braintree respondents with difficulties in coping with the tasks of daily living reported wanting more help with everyday activities or personal care, but more of the Hackney respondents said they would like more help.

In all samples the tasks respondents most often wanted more help with were:

- cutting toenails
- washing self/bathing
- housework
- jobs around the house.

In reply to a question about anything else that could be provided for them that would make it easier to maintain their independence at home, most often mentioned were aids and adaptations in the home (eg grab rails, higher chairs, trolleys and various home improvements).

There were some interesting differences in old people's preferences for who should provide additional help. At follow up, 82 per cent and 88 per cent respectively of the younger and older Hackney respondents who wanted more help said they would prefer this to come from health and social services professionals. The equivalent proportion in Braintree was only 45 per cent. A quarter of the Braintree respondents were unsure about whom they wanted to provide more help while 15 per cent said they would like more help from relatives and friends (compared with 5 per cent in Hackney) and 15 per cent said they would prefer help from private services (compared with 3 per cent in Hackney).

In terms of predicting future demands on formal services, policy makers and planners need to take account not just of friends' and relatives' willingness to provide support, but also of older people's willingness to *receive* such help.

Table 5 Percentage of Hackney 85+ follow-up sample needing help with specified tasks and source of help received

Task	Needing help		% Usually helped by		
	%	Number	Professional	Relative	Friend/ Neighbour
Odd jobs	91	239	30	54	16
Shopping	83	218	47	45	8
Housework	79	207	76	23	1
Laundry	70	184	46	49	5
Filling in forms/writing	65	170	17	71	12
Cooking	43	114	56	42	2
Cutting toenails	67	176	84	14	2
Washing hair	41	109	62	36	2
Bathing	20	53	55	33	12

• Differences in survival

In our research, we aimed to identify the social, psychological and physical characteristics associated with successful survival in the community. Data from the death certificate data collected from the 85+ group allowed us to look at differences in survival from the time of the baseline survey which revealed some interesting variations in the oldest old group. (Deaths in the younger samples are not yet sufficiently numerous to allow detailed analysis.)

Social contact

After allowing for differences in health, the data suggest that men with very few social contacts have higher risk of death than those who do not, while women who belong to social clubs have a better chance of living longer.

Social class

Our research showed that, amongst women, those whose social class (assigned on the basis of husband's former occupation or own former occupation for the never married) was non-manual or skilled manual had a lower risk of death than those whose social classification was semi- or unskilled manual. What is not clear is whether it is relative deprivation earlier in adult life or socio-economic circumstances in late old age that is important – although the former would seem a more probable explanation.

Living with relatives

Many studies have shown that people move in with relatives because of their deteriorating health – which means that those in this type of household are in a sense 'selected' for poor health. We therefore expected to find their subsequent mortality to be high. However, contrary to this expectation, we found the highest mortality was amongst those who were living with spouses at the time of the baseline survey. This warrants further investigation, but it seems possible that among the oldest old, being cared for by an active younger relative may contribute to a longer life.

Gender differences

A higher proportion of women than men were still alive 30 months after the baseline survey as would be expected (Table 6). Amongst men, the most important variable associated with differences in survival was the number of health problems. Those with six or more reported health problems at initial interview had a higher risk of death than men with few problems (Table 7). Amongst women, their score on. the 'activities of daily living' scale (showing their 'functional disability' or degree of difficulty with everyday tasks) was associated with differences in survival – the most able having the highest survival rate (Table 7).

Table 6 Baseline distribution and survival to thirty months follow up of the Hackney 85+ sample by age and sex

	Distribution (%) at baseline		% Alive at 30 months follow up	
	M	F	M	F
85–89	79	73	59	73
90+	21	27	62	70
85+	100	100	60	72
N	136	484	81	348

A more complex analysis of the data, taking into account the interaction of different factors, suggests that among women, increasing age, a high rate of functional disability and belonging to semi- or unskilled manual social classes were associated with an increased risk of death.

Table 7 Baseline distribution and survival to thirty months follow up of the Hackney 85+ sample by sex and indicators of health status

	Distribution (%) at baseline*		% Alive at 30 months follow up	
	M	F	M	F
ADL Score				
Good	43	27	75	83
Fair	39	33	48	70
Poor	16	37	60	65
Health problems				
0–3	48	41	68	74
4–5	31	28	64	70
6–10	21	29	35	71
GHQ Status				
'Non-case'	69	61	61	74
Case	27	24	56	70

* *May not sum to 100 because of non-response to some items*

Quality of life

The overall factors that we consider important for quality of life appear to be associated with survival: the ability to carry out tasks of daily living, physical and mental health status and class. Psycho-social factors such as reported life satisfaction and loneliness appear to have a fairly minor role in terms of survival, although of course they may be essential for emotional well-being. An important question we sought to answer was: 'what proportion of older people had multiple problems or, by contrast, enjoyed good health in the fullest sense'? We approached this issue by looking at the distribution of survey members by the total number of 'good' or 'poor' scores on the eight (or nine in the 85+ study) variables identified as indicators of aspects of well-being (see p 28). Figures 7 and 8 show the distribution of the older Hackney sample by the number of 'good' and 'poor' scores on these measures. In Figure 7, which shows the distribution of the sample by the number of good scores, those with the highest scores have the best 'quality of life', as measured here. In

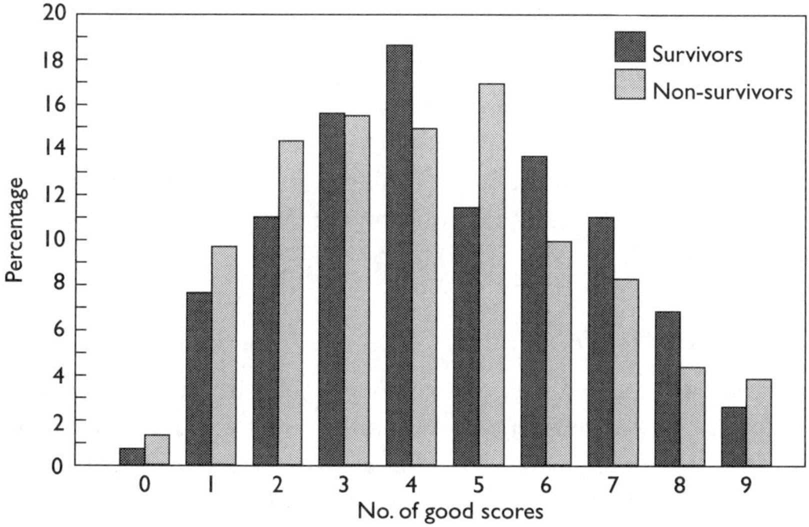

Figure 7 Number of 'good' scores (at baseline stage) among Hackney 85+, survivors and non-survivors

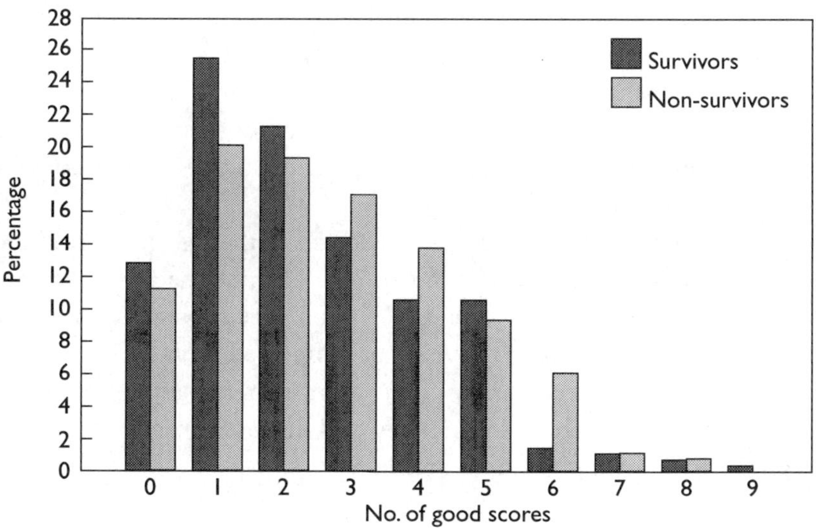

Figure 8 Number of 'poor' scores (at baseline stage) among Hackney 85+, survivors and non-survivors

Figure 8, conversely, the higher the score the **worse** the respondent's circumstances. Those who survived to the follow-up interview are shown separately from non-survivors. It can be seen that very few of the old people had **no** 'good' scores or seven or more 'poor' scores. Overall half the men and 40 per cent of the women had at least five 'good' scores at the time of the baseline survey. The figures also show a relationship between these indicators of overall 'quality of life' and survival until the follow-up stage.

Location and well-being

The results of the two studies of 65–84 year olds in Hackney and Essex suggest a marked difference between the two areas in overall quality of life in these age groups. Those in Hackney were less satisfied with their locality: only 62 per cent like the area they lived in, compared with 90 per cent in Essex. Higher proportions of those living in Essex reported being satisfied with life and they also appeared to be more active.

In both areas, including the older Hackney sample, fewer women than men scored well in their ability to carry out tasks of daily living and more women had fears about opening the door or going out. Fears were higher in the inner city area: over half of those in Hackney were concerned about intruders and feared going out alone, compared with only 28 per cent in Essex.

These differences are, of course, reflected in the distribution of the Hackney and Essex samples by the number of 'good' and 'poor' scores which, as shown in Figures 9 and 10, varied very substantially. Fewer of the Hackney respondents have six or more good scores (Figure 9); in short, fewer had a good 'quality of life' as measured using this method. Conversely, more of those in Hackney had three or more 'poor' scores (Figure 10) indicating multiple problems.

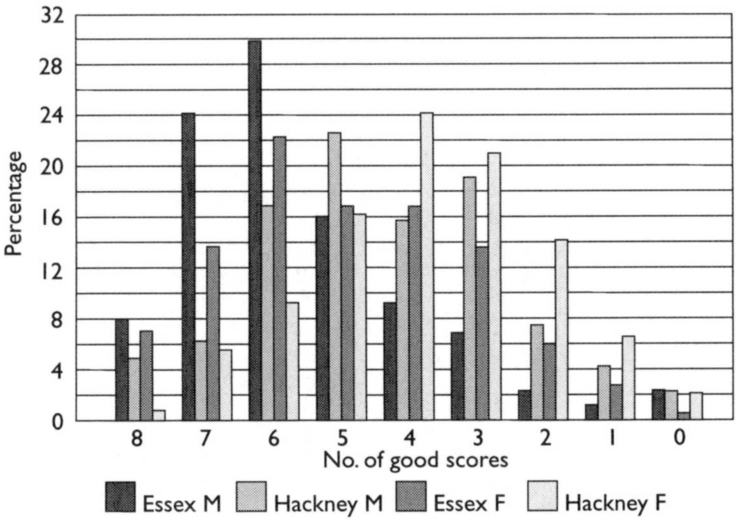

Figure 9 Distribution of males and females in Essex and Hackney by the number of 'good' scores

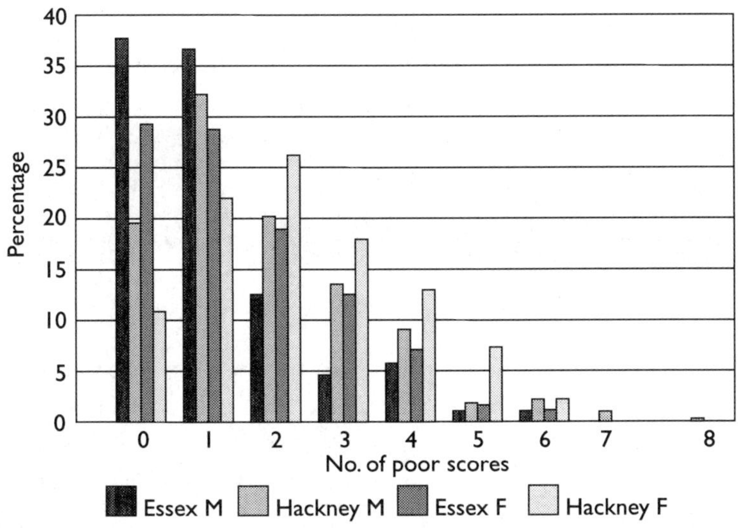

Figure 10 Distribution of males and females in Essex and Hackney by the number of 'poor' scores

4 *What sustains well-being and quality of life in the oldest old?*

In this chapter we examine changes in the distribution of 'good' and 'poor' scores between the baseline and follow-up surveys. We also focus in more detail on those who seemed to have a particularly good or a particularly poor quality of life. The numbers concerned are small and results must be regarded as tentative. However, a similar qualification applies to many existing studies which have attempted to distinguish 'successful' from 'normal' ageing.

By focusing on the small proportion who appeared to have a very poor quality of life, we hoped to identify how early intervention could prevent a deterioration in well-being for older people.

• People over 85 who reported a poor quality of life

Even in the 85+ group, the proportion of people who reported a poor quality of life was small. Only 12 women and one man had poor scores on seven or more of the nine variables (see p 28).

Levels of disability and the number of health problems were, of course, high in this group. Most noticeably all were well above the threshold for needing help with anxiety and depression. Many of the questionnaires also contained other indicators of their depressed mood.

The worst things about being your age

Response to a question on 'the worst things about being your age' included comments such as:

- 'Nobody wants you … nobody likes old people'
- 'Knowing I'm going to die'
- 'I'm a living corpse, I want to die'.

Most replied 'nothing' when asked 'what were the best things about being your age?' One positive response referred to eligibility for entering an old people's home. Despite these indications of clinical depression, only one of the 13 was taking prescribed anti-depressant medication.

Adverse life events

Those reporting a poor quality of life had experienced more adverse life events, such as deaths of close relatives, attacks or robberies in the previous 12 months.

Social network size

The size of social networks was smaller on average than that of the 'good' quality of life group. But it is important to note that, in spite of this, reported levels of practical and emotional support received by the 'poor' group were high. All, bar one, had frequent home help and/or meals on wheels and most also received assistance from home nurses or bathing aides. Five lived in warden-assisted sheltered housing. Twelve of the 13 felt that someone cared about them and understood them and only one reported the lack of someone who would help if needed.

Feeling lonely

A very much higher proportion of this group reported feeling lonely 'most of the time'.

Feeling old

More people in this group reported feeling old in response to a question about whether they felt young, middle aged or old.

Fears for personal safety

Amongst women, the fear of intruders and of going out was important. This issue was brought home to us in several of the focus group discussions when it became clear that most participants lived under curfew conditions, which in winter meant being home before 4.00 pm. Many housebound respondents expressed a wish for occasional outings in a car.

People who reported a good quality of life

The 21 individuals who reported a good quality of life were much healthier than the rest of the sample. They had fewer problems with carrying out the activities of daily living, had a lower than average age than the sample as a whole, reported high levels of satisfaction with life, and depression and anxiety were low. They also included a higher proportion of men than those in the 'poor' group (although this difference was not statistically significant).

These respondents reported high levels of emotional support from family and friends; all had someone they felt cared about them and understood them and someone they could turn to for help.

Five had weekly or twice-weekly home help and several had chiropody – but most made no or very little use of formal services. While those in the 'poor' group reported very few pastimes or activities, nearly all of these respondents reported being involved in regular activities, went on outings or had hobbies, including gardening, DIY, crafts or, in one case, betting on horses. As none of this group was housebound, their opportunities for visits and outings were much greater, but their state of mind and attitude to life may also have contributed to their level of activity.

We were struck by how many of the oldest respondents in good physical and mental shape had outgoing personalities and a strong commitment to making other people's lives brighter and better. The questionnaires completed by these respondents indicated a positive and contented attitude. None of them felt old and over half felt 'young'.

The best things about being your age

When asked about the 'best things about being your age' comments included:

- 'I have time to do what I want'
- 'I'm happy to be alive'
- 'You can do what you want, I like my independence'
- 'I think it's wonderful'.

Changes in the number of 'good' and 'poor' scores between baseline and follow-up interviews

Figures 11 and 12 show the distribution of changes in the number of 'good' and 'poor' scores between the baseline and follow-up interviews (obviously for survivors only). While there was a shift towards fewer 'good' and more 'poor' scores, for most individuals this was fairly slight. It is also worth noting that there were respondents who 'improved', as well as those who 'deteriorated' (although the latter group was larger).

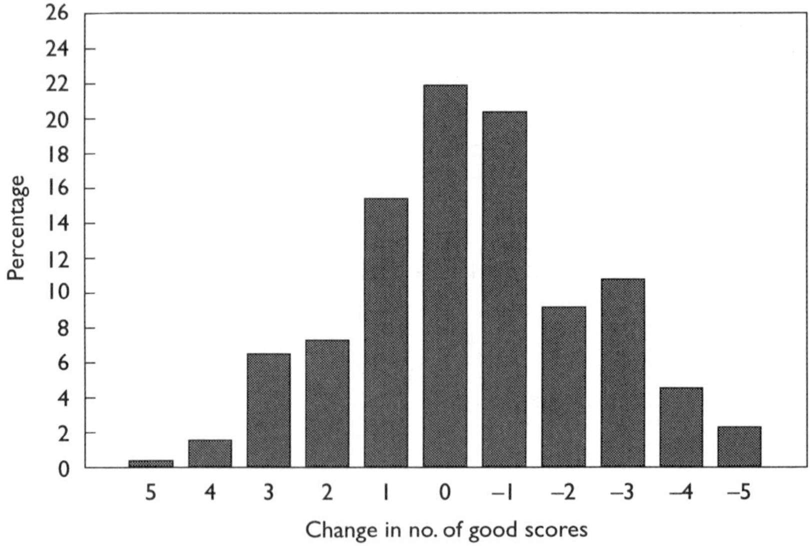

Figure 11 Distribution (%) of the Hackney 85+ sample by changes in the number of 'good' scores between baseline and follow up

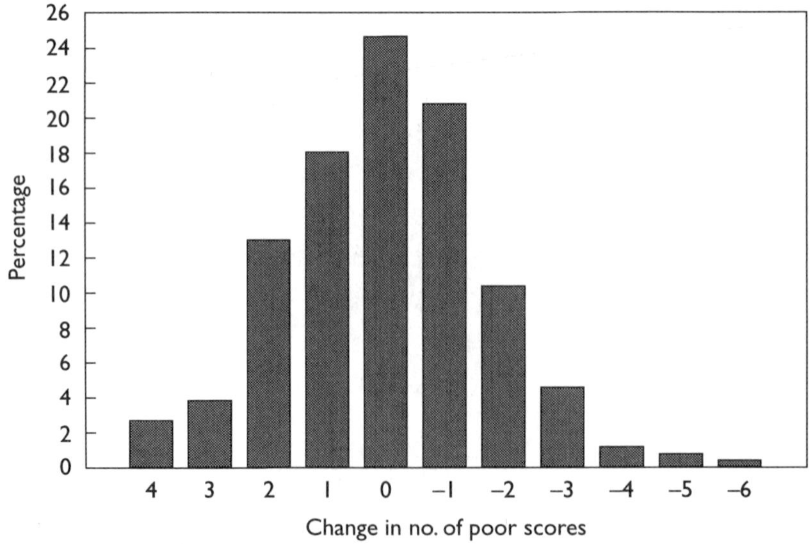

Figure 12 Distribution (%) of of the Hackney 85+ sample by changes in the number of 'poor' scores between baseline and follow up

5 *Implications for policy development and service delivery*

This research was completed before the implementation of the NHS and Community Care Act 1990. It is possible that the consequent introduction of more needs-based assessments has led to greater needs-based provision. However, if these changes have led to services being targeted at those with greatest needs – the most frail old people – it is possible that this has increased the tendency, witnessed in this study, for services to concentrate on maintenance rather than prevention and rehabilitation.

The main focus of this research has been on identifying the factors that help to make old age a positive experience. Our research suggests that some factors may be hard to change in the short term. Indeed, some changes are beyond the scope of service delivery and have more bearing on global social and economic issues. For example, socio-economic status was associated with the survival rates of women in particular, which suggests that experiences in earlier years can affect the quality of life in old age. However, purchasers and providers of health and social care will still be aware that the greater level of need demonstrated within the inner city area of Hackney, compared to the semi-rural area of Braintree, suggests that a concentration of services is important in deprived inner-city areas.

So what can be done to enable more old people to report feeling satisfied with life and to have a better quality of life? This research found a clear association between poor physical health and poor mental health. The implication of this link is that earlier detection of certain treatable problems (such as problems with eyesight and hearing, problems with feet, and arthritis) might lead to reductions in depression and anxiety and an increase in life satisfaction for very old people. Earlier detection of symptoms of depression would also permit earlier intervention and treatment.

Factors that indicate poor quality of life	**Possible interventions to improve quality of life**
Poor physical health Inability to carry out tasks of daily living without help	Early detection and prevention of physical health
Poor mental health Experiencing more adverse life events, such as bereavement, attack or robbery	Preventing and treating depression
Feeling lonely Reduced level of, or no, social activity Few or no hobbies	Developing social activities
Fear of intruders and of going out (especially women)	Improving safety and access
Smaller social networks	Researching the people who need help Supporting families and carers
Feeling old	Encouraging positive attitudes to old age

Maintaining a high level of functioning (the ability to cope with everyday tasks and to get out of the house) is essential for independent living in the community. Once an older person starts to have problems with activities of daily living, all kinds of complications can set in. The less a person is able to get out, the smaller their social networks become the less they are able to engage in social activities, possibly increasing the risk of depression.

• Early detection and prevention of physical health problems

Functional health, the ability to cope with daily living, was the key factor in surviving successfully in the community. Decline in health and functional ability was the strongest predictor of depression and worsening of depression over time and was similarly associated with low life satisfaction.

Maintaining and improving good levels of functioning and activity is crucial for a 'positive' old age. This can be achieved by changing the emphasis of health care for older people away from maintenance and towards positive intervention. The development of rehabilitative services might prevent or delay the onset of serious disability. Given the importance of problems with feet, it would seem that chiropody services are particularly needed, as well as physiotherapy and occupational therapy.

Preventing and treating depression

Our study found that a high proportion of older people were suffering symptoms of depression, but very few were receiving any treatment or help. In addition, many old people said that, although they consulted the GP with physical health problems, they were less likely to do so with symptoms of anxiety or depression. This points again to the need for health and social service professionals to be trained to look out for signs and symptoms of depression and to be alerted to the higher risk of depression after recent adverse life events.

• Social activities: safety and access

Many of the oldest old in our study were unable to leave the house. Other old people were restricted in getting out and engaging in activities outside the home. Our research showed that isolated men have a higher risk of death than those who are not isolated and, amongst women, those who belonged to social clubs had a better chance of living longer.

There was a huge difference between the Essex and Hackney samples in satisfaction with the locality and in fears about going out. Women living in the inner city were particularly worried about intruders and about going out alone. Some were living under a self-imposed curfew, which meant staying indoors after 4.00 pm in winter.

These findings suggest that older people's quality of life might be improved by:

- developing a range of social, recreational and educational activities that are accessible and suitable for old people to enable them to maintain an active life and wide social networks
- ensuring that people have the transport and help they need in order to take part in such activities and to get out to visit friends and family
- crime-prevention strategies in inner cities.

• Supporting families and carers

Our research showed that most old people did have someone they could turn to for help, usually a relative. Relatives, rather than professionals or friends, were providing most of the practical help but professionals were important in providing help with a number of key tasks, such as cutting toenails. With increasing age, older people's networks tended to become weaker with fewer surviving relatives. This indicates that the care of most of these older people is being provided by a smaller number of people (or often just one) as there are fewer people in the network to share the care.

The negative image of very old people as disabled, restricted, unhealthy and unhappy persists, as does the notion that families no longer care for their older relatives. Although our research has highlighted some of the problems associated with old age, it has also shown that many people were in fact enjoying a good quality of life, had high levels of life satisfaction and enjoyed a high level of support from relatives and friends.

References

Measurement of life satisfaction (1966) B L Neugarten, R J Havighurst and S S Tobin, in *Journal of Gerontology*, **16** 134–143.

OPCS Surveys of Disability in Great Britain Report 1 (1988) J Martin, H Meltzer, and D Eliot, HMSO, London.

Predicting satisfaction with social support from social network structure (1983) J P Stokes in *American Journal of Community Psychology*, **11** 141–152.

Social Indicators of Well-Being – Americans' Perceptions of Life Quality (1976) F M Andrews and S B Withey, Plenum Press, New York.

Successful ageing: Perspectives from the Behavioural Sciences (1993) P M Baltes and M M Baltes (eds) Cambridge University Press, New York.

A User's Guide to the General Health Questionnaire (1988) D P Goldberg and P Williams, NFER-Nelson, Windsor.

Appendix 1 Measures used in surveys

These were the scales used to measure different aspects of quality of life and well being in older people.

Functional ability

The functional ability scale was based on questions about respondents' degree of difficulty with a list of 23 activities of daily living (ADL) relating to personal care (washing, dressing and so on), domestic tasks (cooking, shopping, laundry) and mobility (eg getting in/out of bath, going up/down steps, getting about indoors, getting outdoors). The questions were phrased to measure ability rather than performance. Those who reported any difficulty were then asked whether they received any help with this, and if so, who from and how often. The score ranges from 23 to 138, with higher scores indicating poorer functional ability. In some of the analyses reported here, these were grouped into bands indicating good, medium or poor ability.

Social networks

Respondents were asked about all regular contacts and these were charted on a social network grid. This was supplemented with questions on perceptions of the social network's supportiveness (Stokes 1983). In addition, questions about who helped, frequency of help and need for more help were asked on the activities of daily living scale

Psychiatric morbidity

The 28-item version of the General Health Questionnaire (GHQ) (Goldberg and Williams 1988) was selected to measure psychiatric morbidity. This measure was chosen because it has the advantage over depression self-report symptom scales of concentrating on broad components of non-psychotic psychiatric morbidity (eg anxiety and depression, apathy and agitation). It also permits analyses within subcategories and has good reliability and validity. Respondents indicate on a 4 point scale the extent to which items reflect their usual mental or emotional state. Scores range from 0 to 28. Threshold scores on the scale are set to correspond with a 'case' definition equivalent to the average patient referred to psychiatrists. The recommended threshold score is four or five; the higher value of five was used in the analyses reported here in order to exclude the false positive cases as far as possible. The proportion of respondents with scores above the threshold represents the probable prevalence of psychiatric morbidity.

Life satisfaction

Overall life satisfaction was measured using Neugarten's Life Satisfaction Scale (Neugarten *et al.*, 1966), which is a well tested scale consisting of 20 statements presented on cards to respondents who sort them into piles – agree, disagree and uncertain. Scores range from 0 to 20 with the higher the score the better the life satisfaction. Most published studies report average life satisfaction in older people of between 12 and 14. Current life satisfaction was measured with items from Andrews and Withey's Delighted–Terrible Faces Scale (1976), which requires respondents to pick a face (with expressions from delighted, neutral to terrible) to represent their feelings, with low scores representing good life satisfaction.

Mental 'confusion'

Six per cent of respondents living in Hackney who were aged 65–75 and six per cent of those aged 75–85 were rated as mentally confused by interviewers, as were 11 per cent of those over 85, using a standard checklist of items (address, date etc). In Braintree, two per cent of those aged 65–75 and nine per cent; of those aged 75–85 were rated as confused. These respondents were not asked to complete the GHQ or other measurement scales. Where possible a brief proxy interview was conducted with a relative instead, but these results were not included in the analyses presented here.

Appendix 2 Publications based on Essex and Hackney longitudinal study results

The publications listed here include only those arising from the follow ups to the baseline studies. A large number of other publications report the analysis of the baseline data. (A list of these is available from the authors.)

List of Publications

Farquhar M, Bowling A and Grundy E (1991). Elderly people in the community: tailoring the service *Nursing Times* **98** (43) 32–34.

Farquhar M, Bowling A and Grundy E (1991). Report of the first phase of re-interviews with elderly people: sample aged 85 living in City and Hackney. Department of Public Health, City and Hackney Health Authority, London.

Farquhar M, Bowling A and Grundy E (1991). Report of the follow up interviews with elderly people. Sample aged 65 < 85 living at home in City and Hackney. City and Hackney Health Authority and King's College London.

Bowling A, Farquhar M, Grundy E and Formby S (1992). Psychiatric morbidity among people aged 85+ in 1987; a follow up study at two and a half years *International Journal of Geriatric Psychiatry*. **7**: 307–321.

Farquhar M, Bowling A and Grundy E (1992). Report of the follow interviews with elderly people. Sample aged 65 < 85 living at home in Braintree, Essex. City and Hackney Health Authority and King's College London.

Bowling A, Farquhar M, Grundy E and Formby S (1993). Changes in life satisfaction over a two and a half year period among very elderly people living in London. *Social Science and Medicine* **36**: 641–655.

Bowling A, Farquhar M, Grundy E and Formby J (1993). Who are the consistently high users of health and social services? A follow-up study two and a half years later of people aged 85+ at baseline *Health and Social Care* **1**: 277–287.

Bowling A, Farquhar M, Grundy E and Formby J (1993). Disability resulting in 'houseboundness': results of a follow-up survey of very old people. *Generations Review* **3**(1) 7–9.

Farquhar M, Bowling A, Grundy E and Formby J (1993). Use for services; needs for services. Results from the East London and mid Essex longitudinal surveys. *Nursing Standard* **7** (47): 31–36.

Farquhar M, Bowling A, Grundy E and Formby J (1993). Functional ability of very elderly people *Nursing Standard* **7** (51): 31–36.

Farquhar M, Bowling A, Grundy E and Formby J (1993). The housebound: identifying changes over time from a longitudinal survey of people aged 85 and over living at home. *Nursing Standard* **8**: 26–31.

Bowling A, Farquhar M and Grundy E (1994). Associations with changes in level of functional ability. Results from a follow-up survey at two and a half years of people aged 85 years and over at baseline. *Ageing and Society* **14**: 53–73.

Bowling A, Farquhar M and Grundy E (1994). Changes in the ability to get outdoors among a community sample of people aged 85+: results from a follow-up study in 1990. *International Journal of Health Sciences* **5**: 13–23.

Grundy E (1994) Live old, live well: social aspects of ageing. *MRC News* **64**, 22–25.

Bowling A, Farquhar M and Grundy E (1995) Changes in network composition among older people living in Inner London and Essex. *Health and Place* **1**(3) 149–166.

Bowling A, Farquhar M and Grundy E (1995) Changes in network composition among the very old living in Inner London. *Journal of Cross-Cultural Gerontology* **10**, 331–347.

Bowling A, Farquhar M and Grundy E (1995) Changes in health and social service use among three samples of older people in Inner London. *International Journal of Health Sciences*, **6**, 1–13.

Bowling A, Farquhar M and Grundy E (1996) Outcome of anxiety and depression at two and a half years after baseline: association with changes in psychiatric morbidity among three samples of elderly people living at home. *International Journal of Geriatric Psychiatry* **11**:119–129.

Bowling A, Farquhar M and Grundy E (1996) Associations with changes in life satisfaction among three samples of elderly people living at home. *International Journal of Geriatric Psychiatry* **11**:1077–1087

Grundy E, Bowling A, and Farquhar M.(1996) Social support, life satisfaction and survival at older ages. Paper presented to UN/WHO/IUSSP/JARC Conference on health and mortality trends among elderly populations, Sendai (Japan) 21–25 June 1993. In G Caselli and A Lopez, (eds) *Health and mortality among elderly populations*, Clarendon Press, Oxford, 135–156.

Bowling A and Grundy E (1997) Changes in functional ability in three samples of elderly and very elderly people. *Age and Ageing* 26: in press.

Bowling A and Grundy E . Eighty five plus in East London. The Stationery Office, London, in preparation.

About Age Concern

Living well into old age is one of a wide range of publications produced by Age Concern England, the National Council on Ageing. Age Concern England is actively engaged in training, information provision, fundraising and campaigning for retired people and those who work with them, and also in the provision of products and services such as insurance for older people.

A network of over 1,400 local Age Concern groups, with the support of around 250,000 volunteers, aims to improve the quality of life for older people and develop services appropriate to local needs and resources. These include advice and information, day care, visiting services, transport schemes, clubs, and specialist facilities for older people who are physically and mentally frail.

Age Concern England is a registered charity dependent on public support for the continuation and development of its work.

Age Concern England
1268 London Road
London SW16 4ER
Tel: 0181-679 8000

Age Concern Scotland
113 Rose Street
Edinburgh EH2 3DT
Tel: 0131-220 3345

Age Concern Cymru
4th Floor
1 Cathedral Road
Cardiff CF1 9SD
Tel: 01222 371566

Age Concern Northern Ireland
6 Lower Crescent
Belfast BT7 INR
Tel: 01232 245729

Publications from Age Concern Books

Money Matters

Your Rights: A guide to money benefits for older people

Sally West

A highly successful annual publication – now in its 25th edition – Your Rights ensures that older people and their advisers can easily understand the complexities of state benefits. Please ring 0181-679 8000 for further information.

Residents' Money: A guide to good practice in care homes

Residents' Money is a guide for people who work in residential and nursing homes who may be involved in handling residents' money, and perhaps in helping them to manage their financial affairs. It describes the legal requirements and suggests approaches and policies to assist residents in managing their own money.

£6.95 0-86242-205-1

Health & Care

Living, Loving and Ageing: Sexual and personal relationships in later life

Wendy Greengross and Sally Greengross

Sexuality is often regarded as the preserve of the younger generation. This book, for older people and those who work with them, tackles the issues in a straightforward fashion, avoiding preconceptions and bias.

£5.99 0-86242-070-9

The Community Care Handbook: The reformed system explained

Barbara Meredith

Written by one of the country's leading experts, the second edition of this hugely successful handbook provides a comprehensive overview of the first two years of implementation of the community care reforms and examines how the system has evolved. Containing extensive background information on the origins of the new system, this edition describes some of the experiences of those working in the field.

£13.99 0-86242-171-3

To order any of these titles, please write to the address below enclosing a cheque or money order for the appropriate amount and made payable to Age Concern England. Credit card orders may be made on 0181-679 8000.

MAIL ORDER UNIT

Age Concern England
1268 London Road
London SW16 4ER

Index